Contents

INTRODUCTION 4

PART I: UNDERSTANDING CELERY JUICE 6

What is celery? 6

Health benefits of Celery Juice 9

Inflammation 9

MINERAL SALTS 10

MINERAL SALTS PART TWO..................... 12

AUTOIMMUNE DISEASE 14

PH 15

AMMONIA PERMEABILITY 16

Symptoms and illnesses that can be aided by celery juice. 18

Misconceptions about celery juice.................... 30

Celery juice detox tips and FAQS 34

PART II: FOUR WEEK DETOX MEAL PLAN.... 47

PART III: HEALING RECIPES 51

Breakfast 51

Overnight Chia and Oats 51

Fruit Overnight Oats 52

Dippers... 53

Detox breakfast bowls 55

Healthy ham, egg, and chips 57

Salads 59

Broccoli and Shredded Brussel Sprout Salad
.... 59

Spring detox cauliflower salad 61

Citrus tender 63

Quinoa Avo Salad 65

Cauliflower and quinoa tabouli bowls 67

Soups 70

Detox Vegetable Soup 70

Lemongrass Coconut Soup 72

Broccoli Soup 74

Beet Detox Soup 76

Sweet Potato Detox Soup 78

Vegan and Vegetarian 80

Korean bbq style cauliflower lettuce wraps 80

Healthy Pesto Pasta 82

Stuffed Bell Peppers 84

Stuffed Tomatoes 86

Tofu Stir-fry 88

Meats and fish 90

Roasted Salmon Detox Salad 90

Teriyaki Chicken 92

Chicken with Zucchini Noodles 94

Beef Stew 96

Spicy herb halibut.. 98

Italian salmon... 100

Alternative Smoothies 102

Beet it 102

Vitamin C.. 103

Morning Juice 104

Weight Balancing Smoothie........................ 105

INTRODUCTION

Celery juice has become the latest keyword trend in the health and wellness field, and it's making a name for itself as the magical healing cure for a plethora of diseases.
We've seen many trends in health and wellness come and go in the past few years, but what's compelling about celery juicing it's proven itself effective time and time again.

Currently, we're becoming more aware that inflammation underlies many of the world's most widespread diseases, even the process of aging.

Inflammation relates to numerous inflammatory ailments such as rheumatoid arthritis, type 2 diabetes, among others. But did you know that inflammation is recognized as a risk factor for acquiring cancer and heart disease, our most common killers?

Considering the aforementioned, shouldn't we be striving to be more pro-active in decreasing inflammation?

One thing we can all be doing to combat inflammation and hidden pathogens, like bacteria and viruses, is to begin consuming celery juice daily - celery juice is known to combat inflammation and rid hidden pathogens such as EBV.

Let this book serve as a guide to understanding and implementing a celery juicing routine into your daily life. The recipes within each chapter will not only help fight inflammation and viral infections, but they will also work in a symbiotic manner alongside celery juice to better improve the detoxification process.

PART I: UNDERSTANDING CELERY JUICE

What is celery?

Celery is one of the most prolifically versatile vegetables around; whether consumed as a snack all by itself or with peanut butter to enhance the nutrition.
It's advantageous for its flavorsome seeds and green leaves and stalks.

It's a primary descendant of wild celery and a member of the Apiaceae family along with fennel, parsley, and parsnips, maintaining in shape and taste some similar features.
Due to it being a vegetable with high water content, celery demands fertile, moisture-rich soil.

This explains why the plant's origin is thought to be Sweden, Asia, Egypt, and into the Mountains of India.

A vast territory in Punjab is solely committed to celery seed production for exportation purposes into Europe.

Celery is most suitably planted early in climates where the winters get cold, and summers are hot. The more common term for this is cool-weather crop.

Because the seeds are minute, they need to be covered lightly with soil and watered regularly for three to nine weeks; Although another efficient method is starting them indoors and transplanting the plants after approximately two months.

The nutritional profile of celery is incredibly low in calories; it only contains 16 calories per serving.
This is the main reason why it's so popular for people who are dieting.
It is also commonly known as a high fiber food; this is beneficial because fiber moves food throughout the digestive tract at a faster rate, and therefore aids in lowering colon cancer risk.

An interesting fact about this vegetable is the different minerals and vitamins it possesses. Potassium, manganese, phosphorus, copper, magnesium, and calcium are all prime examples in the mineral category, and vitamin C, vitamin b6, niacin, riboflavin, vitamin K, and pantothenic acid, are some of the vitamins present in celery.

Celery is also known as a rich source of flavonoids like lutein, beta carotene, and zeaxanthin, which recent studies have shown to decrease inflammation as well as the risk of heart disease.
These incredible flavonoids are also known to boost the immune system and diminish the growth of cancer-causing cells.

Celery seeds and leaves also contain several volatile oils, such as humulene, selinene, and terpenes.
Coumarins another prevalent component in celery help to thin the blood, and the linoleic acid is an omega-6 fatty acid. What all these and various other compounds do for the body is pretty amazing.

Health benefits of Celery Juice

Ayurvedic medicine has used celery and celery seeds as a treatment for cases of colds and flu, arthritis, spleen, liver disorder, and poor digestion for centuries.

On the other hand, celery juice is a new and trendy refreshment manufactured from the juice of celery stalks, that has been steadily gaining fame and popularity.

The reason for its popularity is because celery juice can be highly beneficial and generates a steady stream of antioxidants and micronutrients that the body needs. Recent studies also show that celery juice can help reduce blood pressure, decrease inflammation, and maintain hydration.

Inflammation

Celery juice is overflowing with potent anti-inflammatory qualities.

This means it's extremely advantageous for anyone who suffers from chronic illnesses, including ailments classified as "autoimmune",

Hashimoto's rheumatoid arthritis, fibromyalgia, Lyme disease, migraines, vertigo, irritable bowel syndrome, psoriasis, gout, bursitis, bloating, intestinal cramping, acid reflux, dizziness, constipation, restless leg syndrome, numbness—all of these illnesses and symptoms are puzzles and their real roots are not yet understood or identified by medical communities and science.

Celery is ideal for reversing inflammation because it starves the pathogens, including unprolific viruses and bacteria such as Epstein-Barr. These pathogens can develop and create numerous conditions and symptoms that normally end up misdiagnosed.

MINERAL SALTS

Celery is capable of starving pathogens; moreover, it comprises several undiscovered mineral salts that function collectively as an antiseptic.

When these potent mineral salts come into contact with viruses, bacteria, and other pathogens, the salts commence to break down the cell membranes, ultimately destroying and removing them from the body.

Celery's potent source of sodium assists in managing blood pressure by raising it when it is too low and decreasing it when it's too high.

Science has not yet undertaken enough research in the sodium components of celery, but ultimately studies will show that these clusters of salts work symbiotically to remove toxins, pathogens, viruses, bacteria, and neurotoxins from within the human body. Furthermore, neurotoxins are produced by viral infections such as EBV living and feeding on toxic heavy metals.

White blood cells utilize these clusters of salts as a weapon to attack viruses and bacteria, which leads to a relief from symptomology.

Mineral salts are vital for the body to function optimally. They keep the adrenals and kidneys functioning and raise the gut's hydrochloric acid so that the body can break down and absorb food and nutrients. They also repair the stomach, digestive tract, and liver.

The mineral salts are building blocks for neurotransmitter chemicals, they kindle electrical stimulus activity, and they promote neuron capacity.
Mineral salts maintain the heart pumping and produce the neurotransmitters required to take information from neuron to neuron.

Celery enhances the efficacy of supplemental GABA and glycine to be assimilated by the body and support in neurotransmitter production for sleep. Furthermore, celery enhances methylation, which is the adequate assimilation and implementation of various nutrients, including zinc and B12.

The electrolytes within celery decrease chances of suffering from anxiety, panic attacks, migraines, and more since these components hydrate the body on a cellular level.

Furthermore, these components also work toward repairing damaged cells within the liver and stabilizing the adrenal glands.

AUTOIMMUNE DISEASE

Celery can break down and remove viruses from the body.
Scientists are currently studying the proposed theory that pathogens such as viruses, including EBV and shingles, are the root of inflammation that's deemed as an autoimmune condition.

The current autoimmune theory is that the immune system is confusing a component of the body for an enemy or intruder and commences to attack it, therefore, producing inflammation.
It's important to know the other scientific theories that are present when talking about autoimmune issues; one of these theories being that antibodies become present because the body is fighting a pathogen that has not yet been detected.

Celery juice is highly beneficial for people suffering from an autoimmune issue, due to the simple fact that celery escorts and expels pathogens out of the body.

Celery juice fortifies hydrochloric acid within the gut. This is extremely important because hydrochloric acid is a vital component for digestion.

When food is consumed, it travels toward the stomach to be digested with the support of hydrochloric acid.
If the levels of hydrochloric acid are low or out of balance, the food that was consumed won't be adequately digested in the stomach. This means that the food won't break down sufficiently for the body's cells to absorb the nutrients, and alternatively, the food will simply remain there and spoil, producing bad acids too.

The rotting in the gut produces ammonia gas, which can travel outwards from the digestive tract into the bloodstream, which can lead to it progressing towards organs such as the brain and liver.
This problematic process is known as ammonia permeability.

Thousands of people suffer from digestive health issues, and one of the main causative circumstances is ammonia permeability.

Another ailment that produces ammonia permeability is a problematic liver.
A stagnant, sluggish, fatty liver produces minimized amounts of bile, which signifies that the body is struggling to break down and disband fats with ease; this also contributes to gut rot, that leads to the generation of more amounts of ammonia permeability.

Celery juice is effective in rebuilding the stomach's intricate supply of hydrochloric acid.
It also fortifies the digestive system by supporting the liver.

Furthermore, celery juice also contributes to strengthening intestinal linings by decreasing the level of pathogens.

Symptoms and illnesses that can be aided by celery juice.

Celery juice has a vast amount of healing benefits for numerous ailments, diseases, and symptoms.

Celery juice supports correct liver function and works as an effective detoxification product.
It nourishes the brain, repairing neurons and refreshing neurotransmitters.
Furthermore, it supports to offset, disable, and expel toxic heavy metals from the brain.
The plant hormones located within celery juice also assist in preserving brain cells; reducing the death of brain cells and serving in the creation of new cells.
Moreover, the hormones from celery juice repair, restore, and enhance the adrenals, supporting and modulating them when they're over or underactive.
Another one of the countless benefits of celery juice is that it alkalizes body and bloodstream, reducing acidosis.

Below are listed some of the main diseases and ailments that celery juice can be utilized to decrease symptomology and eradicate present pathogens.

Rheumatoid Arthritis

The types of joint pain that are experienced in Rheumatoid Arthritis are caused by viral inflammation from EBV.
It has been mistakenly considered as an autoimmune disease, however, EBV is what's producing the inflammation of the nerves and joints.
Celery juice can work wonders for Rheumatoid arthritis because it has extremely antiviral properties, that help expel EBV from the body and decrease symptoms.

Multiple Sclerosis

Celery juice can be an excellent reference for healing when you're coping with multiple sclerosis. You can experience potent healing advantages from it for a variety of reasons.

The root cause of MS is EBV liberating neurotoxins and causing inflammation in the central nervous system.

The sodium in celery juice prevents and expels the virus, minimizing it and eliminating it by eradicating the outer membranes of the cells.

Once the load has been decreased, MS sufferers can obtain respite and relief as their symptomologies begin to lessen.

Fibromyalgia

Celery juice is very beneficial for fibromyalgia because it defuses the toxins accountable for the disease: Epstein-Barr viral neurotoxins.

These neurotoxins berthing on nerves are accountable for the central and peripheral nerve inflammation that is a symptom of fibromyalgia.

When celery juice enters into the system, its sodium content attaches itself to the neurotoxins and carries them outward of the body cautiously. Oftentimes, people with fibromyalgia have extremely toxic livers.

Celery juice cleans and supports the liver, by eliminating several of the neurotoxin infections that the virus generates in the organ even before they get an opportunity to spread to the nerves and throughout the body. With the use of celery juice, overall body discomfort can be decreased, and symptoms can diminish considerably.

Adrenal Fatigue

Celery juice assists any type of adrenal dysfunction by repairing weakened adrenal tissue and damaged adrenal glands, whether the cause was disease or due to a constant state of fight-or-flight.
 Our adrenals are the primary hormone generators, even more so than the reproductive system.

Dermatitis

There are various types of dermatitis, in which EBV is found to be consuming from deposits of copper, pesticides, and aluminum, producing dry skin, irritation of the skin, patches, and dandruff.

Celery juice helps neutralize the viral infection of EBV, also assisting in the removal of pesticides, and the neutralization of copper and aluminum.

Seborrheic dermatitis is more of an effect of a fatty liver, driving someone to generate dirty blood. In this instance, there's no virus associated. It's a liver loaded with a small portion of everything, with toxins leaving the liver and making it to the skin rather than being deposited back in the liver or conducted out of the body.

Celery juice rejuvenates the liver, cleaning out the overload of toxins and enhancing liver cells so that the organ can conduct its over 2,000 chemical purposes.

Eczema and Psoriasis

Psoriasis and eczema are created by a low-grade infection of a herpetic virus within the liver.

Normally, the virus is EBV.

The virus consumes toxic mercury and copper within the liver and then releases them, causing the expelled copper to turn into a dermatoxin.

These dermatoxins travel out of the liver and eventually push up through the skin.

These issues can lead to approximately 100 different varieties of skin rashes, eczema, psoriasis, among others.

None of the mentioned diseases are caused by the immune system attacking itself and the skin.

Vertigo and Dizziness

Some people experience different forms of balance problems.

Some patients experience critical symptoms, whereas others simply feel the room spinning, dizziness, and vertigo.

Furthermore, science is pointing toward the vagus nerve, stating that it has everything to do with the unexplained balance efforts.

Celery juice is one of the most effective anti-inflammatories. It's a potent remedy to support any of these ailments.

Anxiety and Depression

Celery juice assists in finding clarity and happiness.
Celery juice helps to revive the goodness, happiness, clarity, and peace we're all seeking because it immediately addresses the true cause behind mood struggles: toxins. Now, stressful life events and circumstances can create some irritability, anxiousness, and depression on their own. Celery juice can support, because it regenerates the brain tissue, including the emotional centers of the brain, that's where we can convey emotional injuries.

Macular Degeneration
Macular degeneration is produced by a mixture of both toxic heavy metals and viral action. As you've most probably previously

read, celery juice can support both, getting to the root cause of the difficulty.

Endometriosis

Celery juice presents undiscovered phytochemical composite inhibitors to excess irregular tissue development. These inhibitors force back on endometrial mass that seeks to grow outside of the uterus, bladder, and colon. Unusual tissue swelling is due primarily to the residence of toxins. Harmful cells grow and increase where they're not meant to form a sequence of toxic, harmful hormones coupled with agitators such as pesticides, fungicides, heavy metals, and viral or bacterial byproduct. Celery juice tears up and separates all those toxins so they can't feed unusual tissue growth. Coupled with its inhibiting phytochemical composites, this makes celery juice a powerful medicine for people with endometriosis.

HPV

HPV has zero immunity towards celery juice. The virus is comparable in many ways to herpetic family viruses such as EBV, in that its sensitivity lies within the external membranes of the virus, where sodium can connect itself and gradually break down the virus's protection mechanisms. Frequent consumption of celery juice can decrease the development of HPV and defend the cervix from forming scar tissue.
Once you possess the protection—such as celery juice—to combat it, and you're bypassing foods that can supply the virus, you set the tone for defending and even eradicating HPV.

Autoimmune disease

Sodium cluster salts of the celery juice can decrease and expel pathogens, which are the leading reason for the inflammation within the body.

Acid reflux

Acid reflux is a combination of three things occurring; bad bacteria, weakened liver, and decreased hydrochloric acid production. Celery juice aids with these three vital situations.

Sodium cluster salts eradiate bacteria

The sodium clusters found in the celery juice function as a potent antiseptic.
When these make contact with bacteria and viruses, they commence work to break down pathogenic cell membranes, ultimately eradicating them.

Restores adrenals

The vast amounts of sodium located in celery juice support the stability and correct function of the adrenals.

Strep

Strep is culpable for many health conditions, such as acne, SIBO, candida, yeast infections, urinary tract infections, and many more. Celery juice works effectively to destroy and eliminate strep.

Removes toxins from the liver

The sodium and salt found within celery juice can bind onto dermatoxins, neurotoxins, and other viral waste, and proceed by eliminating them out of the liver.

Decreases toxic liver heat

Celery juice cleanses and restores a sluggish liver all the while drawing down the liver heat.

SIBO

Celery juice works as a robust stomach acid replenisher.

This allows for the gastric juices to eradicate strep, which is the leading cause for SIBO. Furthermore, it also helps to eliminate decaying protein and decomposing fat in the stomach and small intestinal tract.
This leads to improvement in bloating and inflammation.

Misconceptions about celery juice

Many people are currently benefiting from this potent medicinal extract, but regrettably, there's also some misinformation, ambiguity, and confusion surrounding the subject of celery juice.

Some of the current misconceptions are as follow:

1. You can combine other foods into the juice.

Celery juice is a potent remedy that is best served and consumed in its purest form. Combining other foods or substances to celery juice, such as collagen, spirulina, or apple cider vinegar, will only disrupt and run the medicinal properties of the celery juice. Accessories will contaminate the purity of this medicine, leading to more limited effectiveness when trying to kill pathogens like bacteria and viruses.

Furthermore, it's not only foods like collagen and spirulina that shouldn't be combined with celery juice. It's also any other fruit, vegetables, leafy greens, and any other type of supplement powders.

2. Celery supplements.

Now there are various products on the market that have become increasingly more popular as more businesses seek to capitalize on the benefits of celery juice.
It's necessary to understand that these products effectiveness cannot replace or be compared to fresh celery juice.

3. Coumarins are toxic.

This is incorrect.
There are copious amounts of research and studies that believe that the coumarins in food may promote the stimulation of white blood cells that protect against cancer.

The coumarins work in a symbiotic manner, that reconstructs, rejuvenates, and restores the complete white blood cell count, such as monocytes, basophils, and neutrophils.

Furthermore, coumarins also support the liver and protect the skin from toxins.

4. Diuretic qualities.

Celery juice has an extremely moderate diuretic effect.
Any food product that has an elevated amount of mineral content will stimulate the system.

Celery juice has a remarkably high mineral content, but its moderate diuretic effect is minimal and necessary for expelling positions and detoxifying the body.

People scrutinize celery juice because the fiber has been extracted and they think the nutrition is lost.
That's incorrect. When it comes to celery, the juice is where the nutrition is located.

Similarly to other herbs, obtaining the juice from celery is considered an extraction method, where the medicinal elements of the plant are obtained.

6. Celery juice contains nitrates.

This is yet again, incorrect.
Celery and celery juice can't carry any nitrates that are dangerous or actuated; the only exception is if the celery has been dehydrated or oxidized.
The commonly occurring nitrates in celery aren't present and don't exist when the celery is fresh and hasn't oxidized.
When fresh celery juice does oxidize, similarly to any other fruit, vegetable or herb, then nitrate can occur.

Celery juice detox tips and FAQS

When talking about the healing properties of celery juice, it's essential to understand that these properties are about pure and unadulterated celery juice.

Furthermore, the full potency of the healing benefits is decreased when celery juice is blended and consumed without straining.

Understandable, celery is healthy, and it's advisable to continue utilizing it in cooking methods and as a snack; but when it's prepared with different techniques the health advantages are incomparable to what celery juice offers.

UTILIZING A JUICER

1: serving

Making celery juice is uncomplicated.

If you own a juicer, here's all you'll have to do.

One bunch of celery

. Cut a quarter inch off the bottom of the celery bunch.
. Wash the celery.
. Put the celery through the juicer, one stalk at a time.
. If necessary, strain the juice to eliminate any stray bits of pulp.
. Drink instantly, on an empty stomach.
. Wait for 15 to 30 minutes minimum before consuming any other meal or foods.

UTILIZING A BLENDER

One adult serving

There is a way of making celery juice with a blender instead of juicing.
If you have a blender, here's all you'll need to do.

One bunch of celery

. Cut an approximately half an inch off the bottom of the celery bunch.

. Wash the celery.

. Set the celery on a regular cutting board and dice into approximately one-inch slices.

. Put the diced celery in a blender and process until smooth.

. Utilize a nut-milk bag to strain the celery, and get rid of the unwanted pulp.

. Wait for 15 to 30 minutes minimum before consuming any other meal or foods.

Rinsing

When utilizing store-bought celery, it's advisable to wash or rinse it before juicing. Celery can be rinsed in hot water, especially if the celery has been stored in the fridge and is chilled. It's recommended not to drink celery juice when it's cold, so washing it under the hot tap will reduce the celery's core temperature by 50 percent, meaning that once juiced the celery juice will be room temperature.

Traditional vs. Organic

When possible, it's advisable to buy organic celery.
If for some unlucky motive it's not possible to purchase organic celery, it's worth mentioning that buying conventional celery is a preferable option to giving up on juicing altogether.
As a precautionary measure, adding some natural soap when washing traditional store-bought celery will aid to get rid of any chemicals before juicing.

Celery leaves are remarkably medicinal.

They are packed with minerals, nutrients, vitamins, and plant hormones.
The taste of celery leaves can be very intense, so if the flavor of celery juice with the leaves becomes unbearable, it's advisable to chop them off before juicing.
This will make the juice more appetizing.

Storing

Celery can remain in the fridge for approximately a week before starting to wither.
It's easy to determine celery's viability by its color. It's important to try and utilize celery before it turns yellow, or brown and commences to lose its green color.

Freshly juiced celery can retain its healing benefits for approximately 24 hours.
It loses its vitality and potency by the hour, so consuming it more than 24 hours after it was made is not going to offer the same benefit or effect.
That being said, if you're unable to drink a full batch of celery juice immediately after

juicing, it can be stored in the fridge, in a glass bottle, with a sealed lid.

FAQ'S

Can women who are breastfeeding drink celery juice?

Celery juice is highly beneficial for breastfeeding. It can deliver a wealth of vitamin C, trace minerals, and neurotransmitter chemicals such as the sodium cluster salts that will help the baby to cultivate healthy organs. Celery juice also supports to purify and detoxify the breast milk, filtering it so that the baby inherits the most unadulterated breast milk.

Can children and babies drink celery juice?

Of course, celery juice is amazing for the development and health of children and babies.

Is it normal to experience stomach discomfort or upset after consuming celery juice?

This is because some people have highly sensitive stomach nerves.

The main nerve that sends signals within the stomach is the vagus nerve, and this system supports the stomach to function regularly. Oftentimes, viral infections such as EBV, create countless amounts of neurotoxins that can somewhat inflame the vagus nerve. Therefore, by commencing to drink celery juice, the juice gets to work immediately and begins to expel the neurotoxins from the nerve endings located within the stomach lining. This process can produce a slight reaction.

Also, it's important to remember that the stomachs of many people are loaded with bacteria such as Streptococcus, E.Coli, and H.Pylori. When these bacteria begin to die off quickly, it can cause slight discomfort or spasm.

Is it ok to consume celery juice while pregnant?

Yes, celery juice is harmless and healthy to drink while pregnant. This matter can be discussed with your local practitioner if you have any worries.

Can I combine ice with my celery juice?

It's advisable not to add ice.
Ice will reduce the healing qualities of the celery juice.

Alternative juices

● Cucumber Juice

One serving

Cucumber juice emulates the equivalent
teaching as celery juice.
This is what you will need to be able to make
16 ounces of cucumber juice.

Ingredients: 2 big cucumbers

Instructions:
Wash the cucumbers and process them
utilizing a juicer.
Drink instantaneously, first thing in the
morning, for the most reliable results.

The alternative method of making cucumber
juice:
Wash the cucumbers, dice them, and process
them in a blender till smooth. Siv with a nut
milk bag.
Drink instantaneously, first thing in the
morning, for the most reliable results.

- Ginger Recipe

One serving

Ingredients:
2 inches of fresh ginger
½ lemon
(16 oz) water
2 tsp raw honey

Instructions :

Shred the ginger into the glass of water and combine the juice of half a fresh lemon.
Allow the mixture to sit for at 15 minutes, preferably longer.
Lastly, add the raw honey if fancied.
Drink instantaneously, first thing in the morning, for the most reliable results.

- Aloe Vera Recipe

One serving

Ingredients:
Piece of fresh aloe vera lead
(16 ounces) water

Instructions:

These instructions are based on utilizing a
medium-sized, bought aloe vera leaf, which
can be found in any major food store.
If utilizing a homegrown leaf, it will probably
possess smaller leaves, so modify the
measurements accordingly.
The most important part is to avoid using the
bitter part of the plant, which is the base.
Start by cutting a section of the aloe vera leaf
open; and then move on to cleaning it by
cutting away the spikes and the skin.
Once the leaf is cleaned, scoop out the gel and
place this in a blender.
Finally, add water to the blender and process
for 10 seconds, until the aloe vera gel is
absorbed.
Drink instantaneously, first thing in the
morning, for the most reliable results.

- Lemon Water

One serving

What you'll need:

½ lemon
16 ounces) water

Instructions:
Press the juice from half a fresh lemon into the water.
Drink instantaneously, first thing in the morning, for the most reliable results.

PART II: FOUR WEEK DETOX MEAL PLAN

Whether you're prepared to commence the healing celery juice protocol, or you're simply curious about all the celery juice hype found on social media, this book and its content will hopefully be of use in one form or another.

Now we're going to jump right into the methods of implementation for the celery juice healing protocol.

First, it's necessary to commit to a minimum of a month of consuming celery juice every day first thing in the morning— while also implementing the other recommendations in this chapter for the duration of the detox month.

Commitment and consistency are the most important factor to consider when preparing to follow detox.

There are usually plenty of issues that need to be addressed within our bodies
 such as rancid fats and concentrated proteins in the intestinal linings; sluggish and stagnant livers, overburdened by pharmaceuticals,

plastics, pesticides, toxic fats, viruses, and bacteria; toxic acidity from the gut to the mouth; high blood toxicity and high blood fat percentage.

Not to mention, the chronic state of dehydration that most people live in without even realizing.

Furthermore, that's not even taking into consideration all the pathogens residing in our organs, bloodstream, glands, and more. Moreover, these are just a few of the basic reasons why it's necessary to allow celery juice to do its job and perform with the highest capacity available. Consistency and commitment are the solutions to a highly potent detox protocol.

Before consuming celery juice each morning during the process of this cleanse, there is the option of drinking lemon water beforehand, the first thing after waking. The advised amount is 32 ounces, and this creates a small liver cleanse first thing in the morning. Before you drink your celery juice each morning during this cleanse, you have the option of drinking lemon or lime water (or plain water) first, upon waking. A good amount is 32 ounces. This gives the liver a cleanse first thing in the morning, which is a great way to commence the day.

By choosing to implement the aforementioned lemon water, it's important to remember that its necessary to wait 20 minutes before consuming the celery juice.
It is advisable to keep in mind that adding water to celery juice or combining the two simultaneously in the stomach damages the juices healing capacities.
If you consume your lemon water and immediately continue by ingesting the celery juice, or vice versa, you will cancel out completely the juice's benefits.
Any time water is consumed before celery juice, its necessary to allow it 30 minutes to work through systems before reaching for celery juice.

These are some of the most important matters to address before commencing the detox protocol.

Meal/plan /days	Mon	Tues	Wed	Thur	Fri	Sat	Sun
Morning Drink	Hot water and lemon/ Celery Juice	Hot water and lemon/ Celery Juice	Hot water and lemon/ Celery Juice	Hot water and lemon/ Celery Juice	Hot water and lemon/ Celery Juice	Hot water and lemon/ Celery Juice	Hot water and lemon/ Celery Juice
Breakfast	Chia & Oats	Fruit Oats	Dippers	Detox Bowl	Ham, egg, Chips	Detox Bowl	Fruit Oats
Midday Smoothie	Morning Juice	Vitamin C	Beet it	Weight Balancing C	Vitamin C	Morning Juice	Beet it
Lunch	Teriyaki Chicken	Pesto Pasta	Roasted Salmon	Tofu Stir-fry	Beef stew	Stuffed bell peppers	Herb Halibut
Dinner	Avo Salad	Spring Detox	Coconut Soup	Detox Veg Soup	Sprout Salad	Broccoli Soup	Tabouli Bowl
Pre-sleep drink	Ginger & lemon tea	Ginger & lemon tea	Ginger & lemon tea	Ginger & lemon tea	Ginger & lemon tea	Ginger & lemon tea	Ginger & lemon tea

Breakfast

Overnight Chia and Oats

Ingredients:

2 tablespoons chia seeds
3/4 cup of oats
1 cup of Cashew milk
1/4 cup blueberries
3 strawberries, diced
1/4 cup raspberries
granola

Instructions:
Combine the oats, chia, cashew milk fully.
Divide into two separate serving
ramekins.
Refrigerate overnight and allow the oats
to soak up the cashew milk.

Top the chia and oats with granola and berries.

Fruit Overnight Oats

Ingredients:

2 tablespoons of chia seeds
3/4 cup of oats
1 cup of cashew milk
1/2 peach, sliced
1/2 plum, sliced
2 basil leaves, chopped
3 teaspoons of hemp seeds
3 teaspoons of pumpkin seeds

Instructions:
Combine the chia seeds, cashew milk, and oats.
Divide the mix into two separate glass ramekins.
Refrigerate overnight and allow the mixture to set.
Finally, top the mixture with basil, seeds, and fruit.

Dippers

Ingredients:

600 asparagus spears
6 duck eggs
Olive oil, to drizzle
Sourdough bread

Directions:

Snap the asparagus spears in half and discard the woody ends.
Trim all of the asparagus spears to a similar length.
Assort the asparagus evenly into six piles, then tie each pile gently into a bunch or bundle utilizing string.

Bring two medium-sized pans of water to a simmer, and add the eggs to one pan and cook for precisely 5 minutes.

Add the asparagus bundles to the remaining pan and cook for 1 minute.
Drain the asparagus and the eggs.
Place one asparagus bundle on each plate, and drizzle with olive oil.
Season with salt and pepper to taste.
Serve with the eggs and bread.

Detox breakfast bowls

Ingredients:

Chai Mix
1 tsp of cinnamon
1 tsp of cardamom
1 tsp of cloves
1/2 tsp powdered ginger
1/2 tsp of ground pepper
salt and pepper to taste

For the bowls
1 cup of cooked quinoa
1 cup gluten-free oats
2 tbsp almonds
1/4 cup of maple syrup
10 of almond milk
1 tbsp instant coffee

Topping
A sprinkle of Cacao Nibs
2 tbsp coconut flakes
cinnamon
2 tbsp coconut cream
gluten-free granola

Instructions:

Firstly, place all of the chia mixtures in a bowl and combine.

Then, place the oats, almonds, and quinoa into a bowl, add the chia mix to the blend and maple syrup. Stir well and set aside.

Heat the almond milk and mix in the espresso shot or the instant coffee.

Pour the espresso milk over the oats, and then place the bowls in the fridge overnight.

Once the detox mixture has soaked and set, remove them from the fridge.

Divide the mixture into separate ramekins.

Sprinkle the top of the bowls with coconut flakes, almonds, cacao nibs, cinnamon to taste.

Healthy ham, egg, and chips

Ingredients:
3 medium potatoes
1 onion, chopped
1 tablespoon of olive oil
400 g mushrooms
4 thyme sprigs
250 g cherry tomatoes
1 tablespoon of wholegrain mustard
4 eggs
125 g ham hock
Chopped parsley

Directions:
In a non-stick roasting tray place the
potato cubes, oil, onion, and a generous
amount of seasoning.
Roast for 20 minutes.
Once roasted, take the tin out of the oven
and add the thyme, and mushrooms. Mix
thoroughly and place back in the oven for
25 minutes.
Remove the tin from the oven and
combine the cherry tomatoes and
mustard into the roasting vegetables.
Then proceed to make four spaces in the

baking tin and crack the eggs into the spaces.
Place the vegetables back into the oven and cook for the remaining 10 minutes.
Finally, top the vegetables with ham and herbs.

Salads

Broccoli and Shredded Brussel Sprout Salad

Ingredients:

Salad
5-6 cups diced broccoli crowns
2 cups shredded brussels sprouts
3 clementines

Dressing
Juice of 1 lemon
Juice of 2 limes
3 tablespoons of tahini
2 tablespoons of tamari
1 tablespoon of pure maple syrup
1/2 tsp turmeric
3 tablespoon of olive oil

Instructions:

Steam the diced broccoli for about 5-6 minutes, until somewhat tender, but crunchy.

Meanwhile, mix all of the dressing
ingredients in a bowl.
When finished, set the steamed broccoli,
brussels sprouts, and clementine into a bowl.
Add the dressing to the salad.

Spring detox cauliflower salad

Ingredients:

Salad
1 can of chickpeas, drained and washed
chili powder, salt, and pepper
1 cauliflower, cut into florets
1 apple, sliced
1 shallot, sliced
a handful of mint and parsley, chopped
2 avocados, cut into chunks

Dressing
2 tablespoons grainy mustard
3 tablespoons honey
1/4 cup extra virgin olive oil
1/2 cup water
juice and zest of a lime
salt and pepper, to taste

Instructions:

Chickpeas:
Preheat the oven to 400 degrees. Position
chickpeas on a baking sheet lined with paper.
Spray with olive oil and add chili powder,
salt, and pepper to taste. Place the chickpeas

in the oven to roast for 30 minutes until browned and crispy.

Cauliflower Prep: Operating in bunches; put the cauliflower florets through a food processor until you achieve a rice texture– it should take approximately 20-30 pulses.

Dressing: Combine and mix all the ingredients in a bowl, then taste and adjust.

Combine all the elements, and drizzle the dressing over the top.

Citrus tender

Ingredients:

Salad

5 cups of spinach
3 cups of arugula
3 scallions, diced
3 blood oranges, sliced
1 navel orange, sliced
1 tablespoon of sesame seeds

Dressing

1 fresh ginger root, slice
1 tablespoon of sesame oil
2 tablespoon of miso paste
3 tablespoons of sunflower seeds
1 Juice of a lemon
1 tablespoon of maple syrup
1/4 cup filtered water
salt and pepper to taste

Instructions:

Dressing:

In a food processor, mix all of the dressing ingredients and blend on high until smooth.
Salad:
Utilizing a considerable sized bowl, layer the arugula, spinach, and orange slices.
Sprinkle the chopped scallions and sesame seeds over the top.
Finally, add dressing to taste.

Quinoa Avo Salad

Ingredients:

Chickpeas
1 can chickpeas, drained, washed
1 tablespoon of olive oil
1/2 tablespoon each of cumin, black pepper, and sea salt

Vinaigrette
4 tablespoons of dijon mustard
3 tablespoons of balsamic
2 tablespoon of pure maple syrup
1 tablespoon of water
2 tablespoon of fresh lemon juice
1 tsp garlic powder
1/4 tsp salt

Salad
1 medium-sized roasted beet, cooked
1/2 of roasted squash, cubed
1 large handful of mixed greens
1/2 avocado, diced
1/4 cup of quinoa, cooked

Instructions:

Roasted Chickpeas: For the crispiest chickpeas, separate all the skins. Lay the chickpeas on an oven tray and sprinkle them with olive oil, rolling them about so they're entirely coated. Roast for 40 minutes until they turn a golden brown color. Once cooked, combine the spices and toss around to coat.

To Make the Dressing. Add all the ingredients for the vinaigrette to a dish and mix until smooth and creamy.
Combine all of the salad ingredients, chickpeas, and beet. Drizzle the dressing over the top to taste.

Cauliflower and quinoa tabouli bowls

Ingredients:

Quinoa
1 cup of quinoa
3 tablespoon of lemon juice
3/4 cup of parsley
3–4 tablespoons of mint
1 tomato, diced
1/2 a cucumber, sliced
salt and pepper to taste

Cauliflower
1 cauliflower, chopped into small florets
2 tablespoon of olive oil
lemon juice
1 tsp of cumin, coriander, paprika,
salt and pepper to taste
3 tsp garlic powder

Tahini Sauce
4 tablespoons of tahini
3 tablespoons of lemon juice
salt and pepper to taste

1 tsp garlic powder
3 tablespoons water

Bowls
olives
red onions
kale, chopped

Instructions:

Cauliflower: Cut the cauliflower into medium-sized pieces and combine in a bowl along with the spices, lemon juice, and olive oil.
Place the cauliflower on baking sheet and roast at 425 degrees for 50 minutes.

Quinoa: Proceed to cook the quinoa as specified on the package.
While the quinoa is cooking, place the leftover ingredients do the tabouli in a bowl.
Once the quinoa is cooked, combine with the tabouli ingredients and mix.

Tahini sauce: Add all the tahini sauce ingredients to a medium-sized dish and blend.
Blend until the tahini reaches a smooth texture.

Prepare 4 containers or bowls. Start by adding a handful of shredded kale and then divide the cauliflower and tabouli. Add the olives, onions and tahini sauce to finish.

Soups

Detox Vegetable Soup

Ingredients:

1 sweet potato, cubed
1 cup carrots, sliced
2 stalks celery, sliced
1 yellow onion, diced
2 tablespoon of olive oil
3 cloves of garlic, crushed
4 cherry tomatoes
1/2 tsp paprika
1 can kidney beans
4 cups vegetable broth
1 kale leaf, chopped
1/ 2 cup parsley
salt & pepper

Instructions:

In a large pot, begin by heating the olive oil over medium heat.
Once the oil reaches temperature add in the cubed sweet potato, celery, carrots, and onion.
Season to taste, and stir well.

Cook the ingredients for 7 minutes, stirring occasionally.

Now combine the garlic, tomatoes, and smoked paprika and cook for a couple of minutes.

Continue by adding in the broth and beans, and place the pot to simmer on a low temperature for 45 minutes, adding water when necessary.

Finally, add the parsley and the kale leaf. Remove from the stove, and let the soup cool for a few minutes.

Lemongrass Coconut Soup

Ingredients:

1 tablespoon of olive oil
2 tablespoons of lemongrass, chopped
1/2 onion, diced
1 teaspoon ginger, grated
3-4 cloves of garlic, crushed
3.5 cups of vegetable broth
3 generous tablespoons of Red Thai Curry paste
Juice of 1/2 lime
1 sweet potato, spiralized
1 zucchini, spiralized
1 celeriac, spiralized
1 can of coconut milk
salt and pepper to taste
basil, shredded
cilantro chopped

Instructions:

Firstly, begin prepping the ingredients, finely chop the onion and lemongrass, and spiralize the zucchini, celery root, and sweet potato.

Continue by adding the olive oil to a pot on a medium temperature, and sauté the lemongrass, ginger, and onion for 6 minutes. Proceed by adding the garlic and cooking until aromatic.

Combine the curry paste, lime juice, and vegetable broth.

Once combined, continue by adding the spiralized zucchini, celery root, and sweet potato.

Lastly, cover the pot, and cook for 5 minutes before adding in the coconut milk. Leave the pot simmering for a few more minutes once the coconut milk has been added, and continue by seasoning to taste and by adding the cilantro and basil.

Broccoli Soup

Ingredients:

2 cups broccoli
2 celery stalks, diced
1 onion, diced
1 cup greens
1 parsnip, chopped
1 carrot, chopped
2 cups of vegetable broth
½ tsp salt
½ lemon, juice
1 tsp coconut oil
1 tablespoon of chia seeds
Toasted mixed seeds
1 teaspoon coconut milk

Instructions:

In a soup pan, heat the coconut oil until it reaches a simmer, and then proceed to add the garlic, carrot, onion, broccoli, celery sticks and parsnip.
Leave to cook over a medium temperature for approximately 5 minutes.
Add the vegetable broth, and bring to a boil.

Once the temperature is reached, cover the pot and let simmer for 7 minutes.

Finally, add in the greens and let them cook for a couple of minutes, then transfer the vegetable mixture to a blender, and add the lemon juice and chia seeds and proceed to process until a smooth, creamy texture is obtained.

Serve with toasted seeds as a garnish.

Beet Detox Soup

Ingredients:

3 beetroots
2 carrots, diced
1 onion, diced
2 garlic cloves, crushed
1 leek, diced
1 tsp of coconut oil
2 cups vegetable broth
¼ tsp salt
1 tablespoon of chia, pumpkin and sunflower seeds
1 teaspoon coconut milk

Instructions:

Start by placing the unpeeled beets in a soup pan, covering them with water and bringing to a boil, then leave the beetroots simmering for half an hour.
Once the beetroots are tender, drain them from the water and set them aside to cool.
Heat the coconut oil in a saucepan, and proceed by adding the garlic, carrot, onions,

and leek. Leave sautéing for 7 minutes over low heat.

Once the vegetables become fragrant, remove them from the pan and place them on a plate to cool.

Continue by peeling the beetroots and chopping them into cubes. Then add the cubes to the blender, and combine with the vegetable broth and cooked vegetables.

Process until a smooth, creamy texture is obtained.

Season to taste and serve with mixed seeds as a garnish.

Sweet Potato Detox Soup

Ingredients:

1 can of lentils
1 sweet potato, cubed
3 carrots, chopped
1 parsnip, chopped
1 onion, quartered
3 garlic cloves, crushed
1 tsp cumin powder
1 tsp turmeric powder
chili powder
¼ tsp salt
2 cups of vegetable broth
½ ginger, grated
1 tsp coconut oil
Fresh parsley

Instructions:

Firstly, turn the oven on and preheat, line a
baking tray with paper, and proceed to add the
carrots, onion, sweet potato, garlic, and
parsnip.
Season to taste, and add the chili, cumin,
turmeric, and coconut oil.

78

Combine all the ingredients thoroughly.
Leave to roast in the oven for approximately half an hour, and then transfer the vegetables to a food processor.
Add the grated ginger, the lentils, and the warm vegetable broth.
Blend the contents until a smooth, creamy texture is obtained.
Garnish with shredded parsley.

Vegan and Vegetarian

Korean bbq style cauliflower lettuce wraps

Ingredients:

Cauliflower wraps
8 cups of small cauliflower florets
olive oil
salt and pepper to taste
lettuce
peanuts, crushed
chives
spicy mayo

Sauce:
1/2 cup of soy sauce
1/4 cup of brown sugar
1 garlic clove
1 slice of fresh ginger
1 tablespoon rice vinegar
1 tablespoon sambal oelek
1 tablespoon sesame oil
1/2 tablespoon of cornstarch

Instructions:

Cauliflower: Combine the cauliflower with a sprinkle of olive oil and a pinch of salt and pepper to taste. Roast in the oven for 25 minutes.
Sauce: Place all of the components for the sauce in a blender and process until smooth. Sauté in a pan over low heat until it slightly thickens.
Empty sauce straight onto the roasting pan – enough to get the cauliflower covered in sauce. Stir smoothly to combine.

Arrange the cauliflower in lettuce cups. Finish with extra sauce, chives, crushed peanuts, and a bit of spicy mayo.

Healthy Pesto Pasta

Ingredients:

16 ounces pasta
Canola oil spray
1 1/2 cups fresh basil leaves
2 cloves fresh garlic
1/2 cup red wine vinegar
1/3 cup canola oil
1/2 cup walnuts
1 1/2 teaspoons salt
1/4 cup fresh Parmesan cheese/ grated
One 4-ounce can black olives
4 plum tomatoes, chopped
1/4 cup fresh carrots, shredded
 1/4 cup fresh red bell pepper, diced
2 cups fresh spinach, chopped

Instructions:

Bring 4.7 liters of water to a boil and add
pasta. Spray subtly with canola oil to keep the
pasta from adhering. Once the pasta is
cooked, rinse with chilled water and set aside
to cool.
Place the basil leaves, garlic, red wine
vinegar, canola oil, walnuts, and salt into a

food processor, and blend on a low setting
until the consistency is smooth.
Place the pasta in a large bowl and combine
the pesto mixture and outstanding ingredients.
Serve warm or as a salad.

Stuffed Bell Peppers

4 red bell peppers
2 tablespoons olive oil
2 cups mushrooms, chopped
2 stalks of celery, chopped
1 cup of brown rice
2 cups vegetable broth
Salt and pepper
One 28-ounce can of crushed tomatoes
1 tablespoon oregano
2 teaspoons basil
1/4 teaspoon cayenne
3/4 cup pecans, toasted and diced

Preheat the oven to 350°F.

Cut off the heads of the bell peppers, and discard seeds and membranes.
Steam the bell peppers for 4 minutes. Extract from the pot, and set to one side. Heat the olive oil in a saucepan over medium temperature. Add the mushrooms and sauté. Next add the scallions, celery, and uncooked brown rice, and sauté for a further 3 to 4 minutes, mixing constantly.

Furthermore, add the vegetable broth, salt, and pepper. Cover, bring to the boil, reduce the temperature, and simmer 40 to 45 minutes, until tender.

Meanwhile, lay the crushed tomatoes, oregano, basil, and cayenne pepper in a small pan. Heat over medium-high temperature, until the mixture starts to boil.
When this occurs, reduce the heat to a low simmer and cook for another 2 to 3 minutes, mixing to combine flavors. Take off the boil and set aside.
Combine the brown rice and the pecans in a bowl. Then stuff the mixture into the bell peppers. Take 1/2 a cup of the tomatoes sauce and spread it across the bottom of a baking dish and place the bell peppers upright within the dish, finally, pour the leftover tomato sauce over the tops.
Bake for 40 minutes.

Stuffed Tomatoes

Ingredients:

Hummus
One 16-ounce can of chickpeas
1/4 cup liquid from the chickpeas
4 tablespoons lemon juice
1 1/2 tablespoons tahini
2 teaspoons garlic, minced
1/4 cup kalamata olives, finely chopped
1/2 teaspoon salt
2 tablespoons olive oil
For the stuffed tomatoes:
8 whole, medium tomatoes
8 sprigs cilantro
8 lemon wedges

Instructions:

Mix the chickpeas, reserved liquid, tahini, lemon juice, olives, salt, garlic, and olive oil in a blender. Process the mixture on a low setting for 5 minutes, oftentimes stopping to mix the hummus. Set aside once the texture reaches a smooth and creamy consistency. Cut a slice off the head of each tomato. Ladle out and discard the centers. Stuff each tomato with the mix, and decorate with a sprig of cilantro. Complete the dish with a lemon wedge.

Tofu Stir-fry

For the marinade:
1/4 cup oyster sauce
1/4 cup soy sauce
2 tablespoons water
1 teaspoon sesame oil
1 teaspoon ginger, minced
1 teaspoon garlic, diced

For the stir-fry:
1-pound firm tofu
3 1/2 tablespoons canola oil
1 1/2 tablespoons sesame seeds
1 1/2 cups peas
2 carrots, julienne-style
1 medium yellow onion, sliced in strips
15 ounces baby corn
8 fresh shiitake mushrooms, sliced
Soy sauce to taste

Set all of the marinade ingredients in a bowl, and mix until well combined.

Drain the tofu and chop into slices. Once chopped, place the tofu in a shallow baking dish and coat with the marinade. Cover and refrigerate overnight.

Preheat oven to 350°F. In the meantime, heat 1 tablespoon of canola oil in a pan on medium-high heat. Sauté the tofu until browned on all surfaces. Return to the baking dish and bake for 8 to 10 minutes.

Once the bake time is over, remove from oven and set to one side.

Heat another 1/2 teaspoons of canola oil in a saucepan at high heat.

Once the oil is hot, add the sesame seeds and sauté until seeds turn golden.

Once again, heat the remaining oil, then add the snow peas, carrots, onion, baby corn, and mushrooms, and stir-fry for 3 to 4 minutes.

Add the soy sauce and sesame seeds and mix all the ingredients.

Put the stir-fry on a serving plate, and top with the marinated tofu.

Meats and fish

Roasted Salmon Detox Salad

Ingredients:

4 wild salmon fillets
1 packet of asparagus
2 bunches watercress
1 avocado, sliced
1 cucumber, sliced
2 beets, sliced
1/4 lemon juice
1/4 cup olive oil
1 tablespoon fresh ginger
1 tablespoon Dijon mustard
1 clove garlic,
Salt and pepper to taste

Instructions:

Place all four of the salmon fillets on the
baking tray, with paper. Continue by adding
salt and pepper to taste.
Bake the salmon for 8 minutes.

In the meantime, cut the ends off the asparagus and cut into cubes.
Chop the watercress, and slice the avocado, beets, and cucumber.
Pour the lemon juice, ginger, minced garlic, Dijon mustard, and olive oil into a bowl.
Season with salt and pepper to taste. Mix thoroughly.
Prepare the watercress, cucumber slices, beet slices, asparagus, and avocado in three salad bowls.
Once the salmon has finished cooking, place a piece of salmon over the top of each bowl, then drizzle with the dressing.

Teriyaki Chicken

Ingredients:

Sauce
⅓ cup balsamic
⅓ cup of agave syrup
1 teaspoon grated ginger
¼ teaspoon ground black pepper
1 teaspoon of miso
1 teaspoon of mirin
1 tablespoon of water

Chicken

1 fill chicken breast
Teriyaki sauce
1 chopped scallion
4 sprigs cilantro, chopped

Instructions:

 To make the marinade, mix the agave,
balsamic, pepper, and ginger in a pan. Bring
to a simmer, then reduce the temperature, and

cook for 15 minutes. Once cooked, let the marinade cool down before adding the mirin, water, and miso.

Marinate the chicken in the sauce overnight.

Heat your griddle to medium heat, before cooking the chicken once marinated.

Wipe away any excess marinade and cook the chicken on the grill for approximately 4 minutes per side.

Chicken with Zucchini Noodles

Ingredients:

1 chicken fillet, sliced in thin strips
2 tablespoons olive oil
salt and pepper to taste
2 full anchovies
chili flakes
2 cloves of garlic, crushed
1 zucchini, spiralized
1 teaspoon of lemon zest
3 tablespoons of chopped basil

Instructions:

Brush the chicken slices with olive oil and season to taste with salt and pepper.

Heat a pan over high heat. When the pan reaches temperature, add the chicken and grill for approximately 3 minutes per side.

In the meantime, heat a normal-sized pan over medium temperature.

Add two tablespoons of olive oil, the chili,
anchovies, and garlic, and cook for 2 minutes.
Continue by adding the zucchini and lemon
zest, and season with salt and pepper to taste.
Cook zucchini noodles until tender.
Finally, top the chicken with the zucchini
noodles, then garnish with fresh basil.

Beef Stew

Ingredients:

1 tablespoon of olive oil
2 cubed fillets of beef
1 can of tomatoes
1 can of tomato paste
2 cups beef broth
1 tablespoon of Worcestershire sauce
1 medium onion, chopped
3 carrots, sliced
3 celery, chopped
1 cup of peas
1 lb. potatoes
salt and pepper to taste
2 tsp. garlic powder
1 tablespoon of thyme
2 tsp rosemary (½ tsp dried)
1 bay leaf

Instructions:

Instant Pot:
Spray olive oil in the pot and turn on the sauté function.

Wait until the pot reaches temperature and proceed by adding the meat, and completely browning on all side.

Next, add the remainder of the ingredients, close the instant pot and turn the setting to "stew" and leave for approximately half an hour.

Once the cooking is finalized, let the stew rest in the pot for 12 minutes, releasing the steam by placing the settings to venting.

Spicy herb halibut

Ingredients:

For the spice mixture:
1/2 cup coriander seeds
1/4 teaspoons cumin seeds
1/2 tablespoon ground red pepper
1/2 teaspoon crushed cardamom
1 tablespoon salt
ground black pepper
Four 6-ounce halibut fillets
1/2 cup flaxseed, freshly ground
olive oil spray

For the garnish:
Several sprigs of fresh cilantro 1 medium
tomato and
1 lemon quartered

Instructions:

Preheat oven to 350°F. Place the spice blend
ingredients into a mixing bowl, and combine
well. Place the mixture inside a pie pan.
Clean the halibut fillets and pat dry. Put
ground flaxseed into an alternate pie pan.
Dredge fillets in the spice mixture first,

followed by flaxseed. Spray the baking sheet with canola oil and place fillets on a baking sheet and cook for 18 minutes. Boil the stock juices for an additional 6 minutes. Pour the juices over the fillets and serve decorated with cilantro, a portion of tomato, and a quarter of a lemon.

Italian salmon

Ingredients:

4 tablespoons extra virgin olive oil
2 teaspoons garlic, finely chopped
2 tablespoons fresh basil, finely chopped
1 medium-sized baguette
Olive oil spray
Four 6-ounce halibut fillets
Salt and pepper
1/2 teaspoon crushed red pepper
1-pint tomatoes
1 1/2 tablespoons capers
4 anchovies, chopped
1/4 cup parsley, chopped

Instructions:

Mix the olive oil, 1 teaspoon of the garlic, and basil.
To cook the croutons, slice the baguette into slices, and spray both sides with olive oil.
Toast till golden brown.
Gently wipe the halibut fillets with the olive oil mixture, and season with salt, pepper, and

red pepper. Place the fillets on a grill and cook, flipping once, until it flakes easily, about 3 minutes each side.

In the meantime, spray a pan gently with olive oil and sauté the tomatoes, olives, capers, and anchovies for 5 minutes, mixing regularly. Add the halibut fillets and lightly spoon the sauce covering fillets until well glazed.

Place 3 croutons on each plate, and top with a halibut fillet and ample sauce. Finish with fresh chopped parsley.

Alternative Smoothies

Beet it

1 serving

Ingredients:
2 big carrots, sliced
1 beetroot, diced
2 apples, sliced
1 celery stick
2 oranges, peeled

Instructions:

Wash all of the ingredients and process them utilizing a juicer.

The alternative method utilizing a blender: Wash all of the ingredients, dice them, and process them in a blender till smooth. Siv with a nut milk bag.

Drink the juice soon after preparing, for the most reliable results.

Vitamin C

1 serving

Ingredients:
5 big carrots, sliced
1 apple, sliced
3 celery sticks
1 lemon, juiced

Instructions:

Wash all of the ingredients and process them utilizing a juicer.

The alternative method utilizing a blender: Wash all of the ingredients, dice them, and process them in a blender till smooth. Siv with a nut milk bag.

Drink the juice soon after preparing, for the most reliable results.

Morning Juice

1 serving

Ingredients:
1 big English cucumber, peeled
1 handful of spinach, chopped
2 bunches of celery, sliced
1 lime
1 avocado, diced

Instructions:

Wash all of the ingredients and process them utilizing a juicer.

The alternative method utilizing a blender: Wash all of the ingredients, dice them, and process them in a blender till smooth. Siv with a nut milk bag.

Drink the juice soon after preparing, for the most reliable results.

Weight Balancing Smoothie

1 serving

Ingredients:
1 lemon, peeled
2 apples, sliced
4 celery sticks
 shredded ginger, peeled

Instructions:

Wash all of the ingredients and process them utilizing a juicer.

The alternative method utilizing a blender: Wash all of the ingredients, dice them, and process them in a blender till smooth. Siv with a nut milk bag.

Drink the juice soon after preparing, for the most reliable results.